Fruit Infused Water
by Neo Monefa

THANK YOU ! CLICK THIS LINK TO CLAIM YOUR 100% FREE GIFT NOW

Table of Contents

9. Mandarin, Basil, & Black Tea Infused Water

10. Meyer Lemon Mandarin Orange Infused Water

11. Orange Pineapple Infused Water

12. Pineapple Mint Infused Water

13. Raspberry Lime Infused Water

14. Blueberry Orange Infused Water

15. Citrus and Cucumber Infused Water

16. Water Melon Basil Infused Water

17. Cucumber Melon Infused Water

18. Citrus Cilantro Infused Water

19. Lemon Lavender Infused Water

20. Honeydew Lime Infused Water

21. Rosemary Berry Infused Water

22. Frozen Fruit Infused Water

23. Strawberry Infused Water

24. Strawberry Pineapple Infused Water

25. Berry, Peach, and Coconut Infused Water

26. Kiwi Infused Water

27. Strawberry Basil and Cucumber Infused Water

28. Raspberry Lemon Infused Water

29. Mixed Melon Infused Water

30. Orange Strawberry and Mint Infused Water

31. Pineapple Ginger Infused Water

32. Cucumber Lavender Infused Water

33. Cherry Mint Infused Water

34. Kiwi, Lemon, and Strawberry Infused Water

35. Cucumber, Lemon, Mint and Rosemary Infused Water

36. Lemon, Lime, Orange Infused Water

1. Introduction

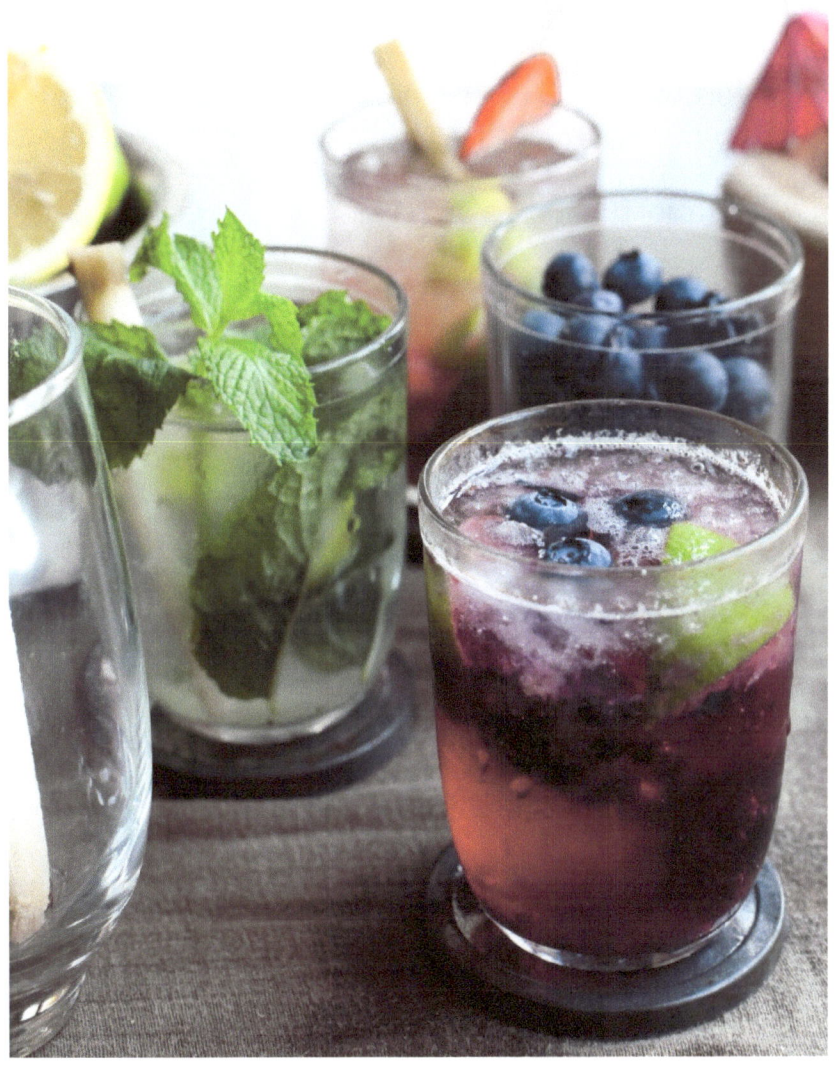

Water is the main component of the human body. In fact, the body is composed of between 55 and 78 percent water, depending on body size. Adequate and regular water consumption has numerous health benefits. As an added plus, it has no calories, fat, carbohydrates or sugar. The amount of water you consume everyday plays an important role in maintaining a healthy body. Experts recommend drinking eight to 10 glasses of water each day to maintain good health. Water helps keep the body well hydrated, which is essential because almost every cell in the body needs water to function properly.

Infused waters can upgrade the flavor without any nutritional drawbacks. You just let the natural fruit and herbs sit in water for a few hours and voila! A delicious, healthy alternative to water. Say goodbye to sodas, energy drinks, and say hello to healthy with these delicious, refreshing flavors! I'm keeping 2-3 flavors of this "spa water" in my fridge now, so I have a variety to motivate me to drink more water.

2. Health Benefits of Water

Relieves Fatigue
If you often feel tired, there is a high chance that it could be due to inadequate consumption of water which makes the body function less efficiently. In fact, fatigue is one of the first signs of dehydration. When there is less water in the body, there is a drop of blood volume which causes the heart to work harder to pump oxygenated blood out in the bloodstream, and other major organs also work less efficiently. Thus, drinking adequate water can help your body function better and reduce fatigue.

Improves Mood
Research indicates that mild dehydration (even one or two percent lower hydration level of hydration than optimal) can negatively affect your mood and ability to think. A small study conducted on 25 women and published in the Journal of Nutrition found that being dehydrated can take a toll on your mood and cognitive function. The color of your urine is a good indicator of your level of hydration. The lighter the color the better the level of hydration and vice versa.

Treats Headaches and Migraines
If you have a headache or migraine, the first thing that you can do to get some relief is drink plenty of water. Headaches and migraines are often caused by dehydration. In a study published in the European Journal of Neurology, researchers found that increasing water intake helped reduce the total number of hours and intensity of headaches in the study participants.

Helps in Digestion and Constipation

Water also improves the functioning of the gastrointestinal tract. This helps in digestion and prevents constipation. Inadequate water in the body often results in constipation as the colon pulls water from the stools to maintain hydration, thereby making them harder and difficult to pass. Drinking sufficient water boosts your metabolism and helps the body properly break down food. This helps your digestive system work well and promotes regular bowel movements. Warm water, in particular, is good for digestive health.

Aids in Weight Loss
In a clinical trial, scientists found that drinking two eight-ounce glasses of water prior to meals can help suppress appetite and hence support your weight loss efforts. When you drink water, it fills your stomach and reduces the tendency to eat more. Plus, it helps increase the rate at which the body burns fat, and promotes the breakdown and elimination of fat cells. Calorie-free water is also a great replacement for high-calorie drinks like alcohol, sugary fizzy drinks and sodas that often contribute to weight gain.

Flushes Out Toxins
Water is excellent for detoxing as it helps flush out toxins from your body and get rid of waste primarily through sweat and urine. It also promotes kidney function and reduces kidney stones by diluting the salts and minerals in urine that cause kidney stones. Though you need to drink adequate amount of water throughout the day, experts warn against drinking too much water (although uncommon still, it is possible) as it may reduce your kidneys' ability to filter out waste. Thus, it is recommended to drink the amount of water your body requires. As the amount of water required by the body tends to differ from one person

to another, it is usually suggested to drink to your thirst, and also include other fluids and foods with high water content in your diet.

Regulates Body Temperature

An ample amount of water in the body also helps regulate body temperature. The thermal properties of water and its ability to release heat from the body when sweat evaporates from the surface of the skin greatly helps maintain an even body temperature. A well-regulated body temperature also will make you feel more energetic when exercising. Water also helps keep your joints and muscles lubricated, thus preventing cramps and sprains.

Promotes Healthy Skin

Water keeps the body well hydrated and improves capillary blood flow, which promotes healthier and younger-looking skin. Water helps replenish skin tissues, moisturizes skin and increases the elasticity in your skin. When the body gets enough water, your skin will feel moisturized and it will look fresh, soft, glowing and smooth. Also, water helps prevent and treat soft lines, scars, acne, wrinkles and other aging symptoms.

Helps Relieve Hangover

Drinking water works as a simple yet effective way to get rid of hangover as well. Being a diuretic, alcohol causes you to pee much more than you take in. Thus, water helps rehydrate the body and speed up recovery. Experts recommend drinking 16 to 20 ounces of water at night before going to bed after you have had too much alcohol.

3. Why It Is Important to Eat Fruit

Eating fruit provides health benefits — people who eat more fruits and vegetables as part of an overall healthy diet are likely to have a reduced risk of some chronic diseases. Fruits provide nutrients vital for health and maintenance of your body. Most fruits are naturally low in fat, sodium, and calories. None have cholesterol. Fruits are sources of many essential nutrients that are under consumed, including potassium, dietary fiber, vitamin C, and folic acid. Diets rich in potassium may help to maintain healthy blood pressure. Fruit sources of potassium include bananas, prunes and prune juice, dried peaches and apricots, cantaloupe, honeydew melon, and orange juice.

Dietary fiber from fruits, as part of an overall healthy diet, helps reduce blood cholesterol levels and may lower risk of heart disease. Fiber is important for proper bowel function. Fiber-containing foods such as fruits help provide a feeling of fullness with fewer calories. Whole or cut-up fruits are sources of dietary fiber; fruit juices contain little or no fiber.

Vitamin C is important for growth and repair of all body tissues, helps heal cuts and wounds, and keeps teeth and gums healthy. Eating a diet rich in vegetables and fruits as part of an overall healthy diet may reduce risk for heart disease, including heart attack and stroke. Eating a diet rich in some vegetables and fruits as part of an overall healthy diet may protect against certain types of cancers.

Diets rich in foods containing fiber, such as some vegetables and fruits, may reduce the risk of heart disease, obesity, and type 2 diabetes. Eating vegetables and fruits rich in potassium as part of an overall healthy diet may lower blood pressure, and may also reduce the risk of developing kidney stones and help to decrease bone loss. Eating foods such as fruits that are lower in calories per cup instead of some other higher-calorie food may be useful in helping to lower calorie intake.

4. Tools for Infusion

Here is the list of things you will need in order to create your own fruit infused water:

Fruit: Just make sure that the fruit you are using is ripe and good. It should be able to provide you with maximum benefits and flavor. Use fresh fruit wherever possible. In case fresh fruit is unavailable, you may want to use frozen, organic fruit. You should also ensure that you wash the fruit thoroughly before slicing and cutting them.

Herbs: Well, herbs are optional and using them depends on your personal preference. A number of herbs are known to complement the fruit flavor in water. Use whatever herbs are available to you.

Knife: You may want to use a small knife for smaller fruits and a longer knife for bigger fruits. Keep your knives clean and sharp to make your job easy and quick.

Jars, Pitchers, and Containers: You really do not have to buy any fancy pitchers and jars unless you really would like to. Any glass jar or pitcher will work just fine. You can use any size container or jar. The thin glasses seem to work well too. Glass is used because it does not absorb any flavors of previous liquids.

A muddler or Wooden Spoon: This is used for mashing the herbs and fruits. It just aids in releasing their flavors into the water. You could mash the fruits and herbs just before adding them to water.

Water: Filtered water is the best; however, you may choose to use regular tap water in case you like the taste.

Ice: Ice is not a mandatory requirement. However, you may choose to use ice if you like your fruit infused water to be extra chilled.

5. Grape Pineapple Infused Water

Grape Pineapple Infused *Water*

Ingredients:
6 organic red grapes, cut into half
1 pineapple spear (3"-4" long)

Directions:
Infuse in the refrigerator for 4 to 24 hours. Longer infusion times will result in a more potent flavor. Serve cold.

Because grapes are not as flavorful as the pineapple, you can use as many as you would like, but 6 works well for this size of container. Be sure to use organic grapes and to cut them in half so that their juices can escape. Bonus: the grapes are still tasty after being infused and you can eat them after you are have finished drinking your water.

This recipe is easy to scale up. The key is to not use too much pineapple because it will dominate the flavor of the grapes. A good rule of thumb is to use 6-8 grapes for every wedge of pineapple.

6. Mango Mint Infused Water

Mango Mint Infused *Water*

Ingredients:
2 sprigs of fresh organic mint (or about 8 small leaves)
1/2 mango, with the skin cut off and divided into pieces (about 6)

Directions:
Combine the mint and mango with water and let the infusion sit for 3-4 hours at room temperature. The warmer temperature helps the ingredients' flavors intensify more quickly. You can also infuse in your refrigerator for up to 12 hours.

After infusing and drinking, you can try to eat the mango pieces. I found that the infusion process had made them softer than when I had started.

7. Cucumber Jalapeño Mint Infused Water

Cucumber Jalapeño Mint Infused *Water*

Ingredients:
3" of cucumber (English or regular), sliced
1/2 jalapeño pepper, de-seeded
1 sprig of organic mint leaves

Directions:
To de-seed a jalapeño, cut off the pepper's top, then cut the pepper in half. Wear a latex glove or cover your thumb with plastic wrap, and run your thumb down the length of the pepper, removing all seeds and the pith. Combine the ingredients in a container and cover with cold water. Infused for 4-24 hours in the refrigerator. Longer infusion times will result in stronger flavors.

8. Strawberry Jalapeno Infused Water

Strawberry Jalapeno Infused *Water*

Ingredients:
3 organic strawberries
 1/4 to 1/2 of a jalapeño pepper

Directions:
Cut the tops off of the strawberries and slice them into two for maximum surface area. Use a plastic glove or piece of plastic wrap over your thumb to de-seed the pepper. Fill with cold water and infuse in your refrigerator for 3-12 hours. Enjoy cold.

Increase or Decrease spiciness: 1/2 of a jalapeño pepper will produce a spicy water! If you typically eat spicy foods, you'll have no problem with the flavor of 1/2 of an infused jalapeño pepper. On the other hand, 1/4 of a pepper produces a very faint spiciness...almost too little to taste. If you have sensitive taste buds, use 1/4 pepper.

9. Mandarin, Basil, & Black Tea Infused Water

Mandarin, Basil, & Black Tea Infused Water

Ingredients:
3 mandarin oranges, sliced in half
4 basil leaves, torn
Black tea bag

Directions:
Combine ingredients with filtered water and infuse at room temperature for 2-3 hours. Pour over ice or enjoy as is.

It's important to infuse this recipe at room temperature because of the tea. Tea does not infuse well in cold temperatures, which is why we are always pouring hot water over it! However, infused at room temperature, black tea is a pleasant, antioxidant-rich ingredient. The infused tea will also contribute a little caffeine, but less than your normal iced tea and certainly less than coffee.

10. Meyer Lemon Mandarin Orange Infused Water

Meyer Lemon **Mandarin** Orange Infused *Water*

Ingredients:
2 Meyer lemons ends removed and sliced,
4 mandarin oranges, peeled and halved

Directions:
Combine with fresh water and infuse for 2-6 hours. You can remove the lemon peel if you are concerned about bitterness. Both Meyer lemons and mandarin oranges are naturally sweeter than regular lemons and oranges, but if you infuse for too long with the lemon peel on or if you find the finished flavor to be too tart, add a teaspoon of high quality maple syrup for a more palatable flavor.

Be sure to cut off the ends of the lemons to avoid the extra bitterness from the rind. You can squeeze the juice from the cut-off lemon ends into your mixture. To peel a mandarin orange or tangerine, start at the top and work your way down.
Next slice each lemon into 3-4 slices. Slice the mandarin oranges in half so that the juice can escape when infused.

11. Orange Pineapple Infused Water

Orange Pineapple Infused *Water*

Ingredients:
1/2 pineapple, quartered
1 orange, sliced with peel on
Top with Ice
Top with Water

Directions:
Fill pitcher or glass with ice and water. For the best flavor, infuse for 2 hours before serving. And when the mixture runs down to the halfway point of the dispenser, simply fill with more ice and water. You can infuse up to three times.

12. Pineapple Mint Infused Water

Pineapple Mint Infused *Water*

Ingredients:
½ pineapple, cut in chunks
4 mint leaves, cut in halves
Top with Ice
Top with Water

Directions:
It's best to infuse pineapple for 8-12 hours. Also, be sure to tear or crush the mint leaves to release their natural oils.
Infuse in the refrigerator for 8 hours or overnight.
Strain before serving but this optional.

13. Raspberry Lime Infused Water

Raspberry Lime Infused *Water*

Ingredients:
8-10 raspberries
1 lime with rind removed

Directions:
Infuse for 1-12 hours and strain before serving.

To muddle the raspberries, simply crush them with your muddler until you see the juice escape. There will be some raspberry pieces in the water as a result of the muddling, so it's best to strain through mesh strainer before serving.

Lastly, it's important to cut the rind off of the lime for this recipe.

14. Blueberry Orange Infused Water

Blueberry Orange Infused *Water*

Ingredients:
6 cups water
2 mandarin oranges, cut into wedges
½ cup of blueberries
Ice

Directions:
Combine all ingredients in a pitcher and put in the fridge for 2-24 hours to allow the water to infuse. You can also squeeze in the juice of one mandarin orange and muddle the blueberries to intensify flavor a bit.
Serve cold.

15. Citrus and Cucumber Infused Water

Citrus and Cucumber Infused Water

Ingredients:
2-3 liters water
2 large oranges, sliced
1 lemon, sliced
½ large cucumber, sliced
 Handful of fresh mint

Directions:
Put oranges, lemon and cucumber in the water pitcher. Using a long spoon   gently mash fruits/veggies; this will release more flavor.

Take the mint, and gently mash it to release the natural oils; add to the pitcher.

Add water to the pitcher, and stir to begin the infusion process.

Drink/serve immediately, or store in the refrigerator for up to 2 days.

16. Water Melon Basil Infused Water

Water-**Melon** Basil Infused *Water*

Ingredients:
2 slices of watermelon, cut into thirds or quarters
Small handful of basil, scrunched
Ice and cold filtered water

Directions:
Fill your juice pitcher to the top with ice and fruit.
Slightly scrunch up the basil so it releases its flavor.
Cover with cold filtered water. This water is best if
you let the water infuse at least 1 hour. If you're
inpatient (like me), poke a few holes in your fruit
with a fork for instant flavor.

17. Cucumber Melon Infused Water

Cucumber **Melon** Infused *Water*

Ingredients:
One large cucumber, sliced
1/4 honeydew melon, cubed
1/4 cantaloupe, cubed
One half gallon of water

Directions:
Place melon and cucumber in a glass pitcher and add water. Allow to rest,
Refrigerated, for two hours and then serve over ice. Garnish with melon
Balls skewered on a swizzle stick.

18. Citrus Cilantro Infused Water

Citrus Cilantro Infused *Water*

Ingredients:
One large lemon, sliced
One large lime, sliced
One large orange, sliced
1/4 cup cilantro leaves

Directions:
Pour water over citrus fruits and cilantro. Refrigerate for two hours. Serve
over ice and garnish with an orange slice and sprig of cilantro.

19. Lemon Lavender Infused Water

Lemon Lavender Infused *Water*

Ingredients:
Three large lemons, thickly sliced
 1/4 cup fresh lavender
One half gallon of water

Directions:
Pour water over the lemons and lavender.
Refrigerate for two hours and
Serve over ice, garnished with a sprig of lavender.

20. Honeydew Lime Infused Water

Honeydew Lime Infused *Water*

Ingredients:
2–3 slices of ripe honeydew melon
1 lime, sliced
4 sprigs of mint
1 half-gallon of water

Directions:
Add melon slices, lime slices and mint sprigs to a large pitcher; fill with the
half-gallon of water and refrigerate 2–4 hours. Serve in ice-filled glasses.

21. Rosemary Berry Infused Water

Rosemary **Berry** Infused *Water*

Ingredients:
1 cup fresh blueberries, lightly crushed
2 4–inch sprigs of fresh rosemary, lightly bruised (to release more flavor)
1 half-gallon of water

Directions:
Add blueberries and rosemary sprigs to a large pitcher; fill with the half gallon
of water and refrigerate 2–4 hours. Serve in ice-filled glasses.

22. Frozen Fruit Infused Water

Frozen Fruit Infused *Water*

Ingredients:
2 cups frozen apple chunks, grapes, or berries
1 half-gallon of water

Directions:
Add frozen fruit to a pitcher; pour water over fruit and let sit at least
30 minutes in the refrigerator. Stir to distribute fruit flavor and serve in
glasses with some ice cubes. (Note: you can chop up the same kind of
fruit, unfrozen, and follow same directions. You'll need to use more ice
when serving the unfrozen fruit–flavored water).

23. Strawberry Infused Water

Strawberry Infused *Water*

Ingredients:
4 sliced strawberries
1 half-gallon water

Directions:
In a large pitcher, add 4 sliced strawberries; fill with the half-gallon of water and refrigerate 2–4 hours. Serve in ice-filled glasses.

24. Strawberry Pineapple Infused Water

Strawberry Pineapple Infused *Water*

Ingredients:
One cored pineapple
One carton of strawberries (sliced)
Ice and Water

Directions:
In a large pitcher, add one cored pineapple and a carton of sliced
strawberries; fill with the half-gallon of water and refrigerate 2–4 hours.

25. Berry, Peach, and Coconut Infused Water

Berry, **Peach**, and Coconut Infused *Water*

Ingredients:
1 cup organic blueberries
1 cup organic blackberries
2 dough nut peaches, pitted and cut into half-inch wedges
6 cups spring or filtered water
2 cups unsweetened organic coconut water
1 gallon clean glass jar with lid

Directions:
1. Place blueberries and blackberries into the bottom of your jar, then the peach slices on top.
2. Pour the spring water and coconut water into the jar. Stir the water, cover with a lid and put water into the refrigerator for at least one hour or overnight for the best flavor. Drink within two days.

26. Kiwi Infused Water

Kiwi Infused *Water*

Ingredients:
3-4 ripe kiwis, peeled and thinly sliced (or crushed for more flavor)
2 quarts filtered or spring water

Directions:
1. Add the sliced kiwis to a 64-ounce Mason jar or pitcher.
2. Add the filtered water.
3. Refrigerate until cold and enjoy.

27. Strawberry Basil and Cucumber Infused Water

Strawberry Basil and Cucumber Infused Water

Ingredients:
3 basil leaves roughly chopped
1 strawberry sliced
3-5 slices of cucumber
Ice
Water

Directions:
Combine all the ingredients in a large glass, and let sit for at least 5 minutes before enjoying.

28. Raspberry Lemon Infused Water

Raspberry Lemon Infused *Water*

Ingredients:
2 cups organic raspberries
8 cups spring or filtered water
1 large organic lemon, cut into half-inch slices
2 dried Medjool dates
1 gallon clean glass jar with lid

Directions:
Place raspberries into the bottom of your jar. Add the dates, then layer the lemon slices on top. Pour water into jar and place lid on top.
Place water into the refrigerator and let infuse for 1 hour.

29. Mixed Melon Infused Water

Mixed Melon Infused Water

Ingredients:
1 cup cantaloupe pieces
1 cup watermelon pieces
1 cup honeydew pieces
2 quarts filtered or spring water

Directions:
Add your melons to a 64-ounce Mason jar or pitcher.
Pour the water over top and chill. Serve over ice.

30. Orange Strawberry and Mint Infused Water

Orange Strawberry and Mint Infused *Water*

Ingredients:
1/4 cup fresh mint
1/2 cup strawberries, sliced
1/2 orange, sliced
16 ounces filtered water

Directions:
Place all fruits and herbs into the Mason jar.
Fill to top with water.
Seal Mason jar tightly and let it sit overnight in the refrigerator.

31. Pineapple Ginger Infused Water

Pineapple Ginger Infused *Water*

Ingredients:
1 cup fresh pineapple pieces (crushed for more a sweeter taste)
1-inch piece ginger, thinly sliced
2 quarts filtered or spring water

Directions:
Add the pineapple and ginger to a 64-ounce Mason jar or pitcher.
Pour the water over top and refrigerate until cold.
Serve over ice.

32. Cucumber Lavender Infused Water

Cucumber Lavender Infused *Water*

Ingredients:
1 cucumber, thinly sliced
1 teaspoon dried culinary lavender, or 2 fresh lavender sprigs
2 quarts filtered or spring water

Directions:
Add the cucumbers and lavender to a 64-ounce Mason jar or pitcher.
Add the filtered water. If using dried lavender, strain before serving.
Refrigerate until cold and enjoy.

33. Cherry Mint Infused Water

Cherry Mint Infused *Water*

Ingredients:
1 quart canning jar
8 fresh cherries, halved
1/4 cup of fresh mint leaves

Directions:
Add the cherry halves and fresh mint leaves to your 8 oz. canning jar. Rip the leaves in half for more flavor. Next, use a spoon or a fork to gently mash the fruit down a little bit. This will let the juice out of the fruit to infuse your water. Fill the jar with water, place the cover on, give it a good shake and refrigerate overnight for the best flavor.

34. Kiwi, Lemon, and Strawberry Infused Water

Kiwi, Lemon, and **Strawberry** Infused *Water*

Ingredients:
4 kiwis, peeled and thinly sliced
1 lemon, thinly sliced
1 pint or 2 cups of strawberries, halved
Top with Ice
Top with Water

Directions:
Add the kiwi, lemon and strawberries to your water pitcher. Muddle gently with a wooden spoon. Top with ice and water. Refrigerate for at least 1 hour before serving. This drink will keep for up to 2 days in the refrigerator or until the fruit turns bad. The peel from the lemon may turn this drink slightly bitter after being infused for over 24 hours.

35. Cucumber, Lemon, Mint and Rosemary Infused Water

Cucumber, Lemon, Mint and Rosemary Infused
Water

Ingredients:
1 Cucumber thinly sliced (peeling is optional)
1 small lemon, thinly sliced
4 sprigs of fresh mint
2 sprigs of rosemary
Top with ice
Top with water

Directions:
Crush the rosemary and mint first before adding the remaining ingredients to your water pitcher. Muddle gently with a wooden spoon. Top with ice and water. Refrigerate for at least 2 hours before serving. This drink will keep for up to 2 days in the refrigerator or until the fruit turns bad.

36. Lemon, Lime, Orange Infused Water

Lemon, **Lime**, Orange Infused *Water*

Ingredients:
1 orange, cut into segments
1 lime, thinly sliced
1 lemon, thinly sliced
Top with Ice
Top with Water

Directions:
Cut each piece of fruit into half and then into small segments. Place the fruit into your water pitcher and use a wooden spoon to smash up the fruit slightly so the juices will flow freely. Top with ice and water. You can drink this immediately but for the best results allow to stay in the fridge from 2-24 hours. This drink will keep for up to 2 days in the refrigerator or until the fruit turns bad. The peel from the citrus fruit may turn this drink slightly bitter after being infused for over 24 hours.

37. Blueberry, Pineapple, Strawberry Infused Water

Blueberry, **Pineapple**, **Strawberry** Infused *Water*

Ingredients:
½ pint or 1 cup of blueberries
½ cup of strawberries, halved
½ cup of pineapple, in chunks
Top with Ice
Top with Water

Directions:
Add blueberries, strawberries and pineapple to your water pitcher. Gently muddle with a wooden spoon. Top with ice and water. Refrigerate for at least 2 hours before serving. This drink will keep for up to 2 – 3 days in the refrigerator or until the fruit turns bad.

38. Ginger, Lime, and Papaya Infused Water

Ginger, Lime, and Papaya Infused *Water*

Ingredients:
1 cup of papaya, peeled, deseeded and cut into chunks
1 lime, thinly sliced
2 inches of ginger root, peeled and thinly sliced
Top with Ice
Top with Water

Directions:
Add the papaya, lime and ginger to a water pitcher. Muddle gently with a wooden spoon. Top with ice and water. Refrigerate for at least 2 hours before serving. This drink will keep for up to 2 days in the refrigerator or until the fruit turns bad. The peel from the lime may turn this drink slightly bitter after being infused for over 24 hours.

39. Basil, Cucumber and Lemon Infused Water

Basil, **Cucumber** and Lemon Infused *Water*

Ingredients:
1 cucumber, thinly sliced
1lemon, halved then cut into small segments
20 basil leaves, ripped
Top with Ice
Top with Water

Directions:
Add cucumber, lemon and basil leaves to your pitcher. Muddle with a wooden spoon. Top with ice and water. Refrigerate for at least 1 hour. This drink will keep for up to 2 days in the refrigerator or until the fruit turns bad. The peel from the citrus fruit may turn this drink slightly bitter after being infused for over 24 hours.

40. Apple, Blueberry, and Plum Infused Water

Apple, Blueberry, and **Plum** Infused *Water*

Ingredients:
2 apples, cored and cut into small segments
½ pint or 1 cup of blueberries
2 plum, pitted and cut into small segments
Top with Ice
Top with Water

Directions:
Add the apples, blueberries and plums to your water pitcher. Gently muddle with a wooden spoon. Top with ice and water. Refrigerate for at least 1 hour before serving. This infusion also tastes great if you add some mint or sage to the mixture. This drink will keep for up to 2 days in the refrigerator.

41. Kiwi and Strawberry Infused Water

Kiwi and **Strawberry** Infused *Water*

Ingredients:
4 kiwis, peeled and thinly sliced
8 strawberries, quartered
Top with Ice
Top with Water

Directions:
Add kiwis and strawberries to a water pitcher. Muddle with a wooden spoon without pulverizing the fruit. Top with ice and water and refrigerate for at least 2 hours before serving. This drink will keep for up to 2 days in the refrigerator.

42. Honeydew and Strawberry Infused Water

Honeydew and **Strawberry** Infused *Water*

Ingredients:
1 Cup of honeydew cubes
2 cups of sliced fresh strawberries
Top with Water
Top with Ice

Directions:
Top with ice and water and refrigerate for at least 2 hours before serving. This drink will keep for up to 2 days in the refrigerator.

43. Tropic Orange and Mango Infused Water

Tropic **Orange** and **Mango** Infused *Water*

Ingredients:
1 orange (peeled and thinly sliced)
1 ripe mango (peeled and thinly sliced)
Top with Ice
Top with Water

Directions:
Place the sliced orange and mango pieces in a glass or pitcher. Pour the water in the container. Add ice if preferred. Chill in the refrigerator for at least 2 hours. Serve and enjoy.

44. Conclusion

Again, thank you for downloading this book. I hope that this book can become an instrument that can help you change your lifestyle and become fit. I also hope you have enjoyed creating these quick, easy, and healthy spa inspired vitamin water recipes.

Now that you have gained more knowledge about fruit infused water, you are in a better position to change your life for the better. This is your opportunity to also help your friends and family members lead a healthier lifestyle. You can share with them the valuable information and recipes you have learned in this book so they too can live a more healthy and fit life.

Step out into a new and improved you with the tips and resources you have gained. Good Luck.

THANK YOU ! CLICK THIS LINK TO CLAIM YOUR 100% FREE GIFT NOW

www.ingramcontent.com/pod-product-compliance
Lightning Source LLC
Chambersburg PA
CBHW050752290526
45792CB00008B/2144